Table of Contents

Legal Disclaimer

While every attempt has been made to ensure that the information presented here is correct, the contents herein are a reflection of the views of the author and are meant for educational and informational purposes only. This book is for information purposes only and are not warranted for content, accuracy or any other implied or explicit purpose.

The author shall in no event be held liable for any loss or other damages, including but not limited to special, incidental, consequential or other damages.

Introduction

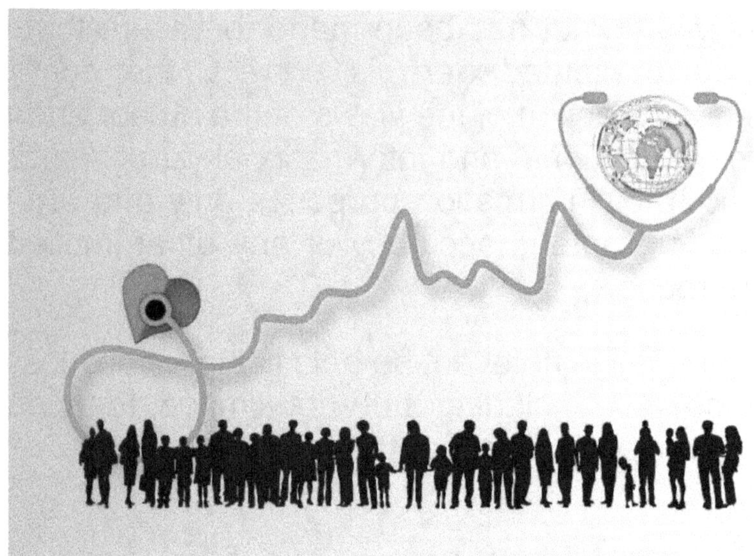

Heart attack is one of the most common causes of death in the world. With most of us suffering from various health problems and putting a lot of extra stress on our hearts due to inactivity and bad eating habits, it's no wonder that many of us are ticking time bombs before we experience it. the heart attack itself.

Mother Nature took hundreds of thousands of years of evolution to develop your heart along with the rest of your body.

Perfect in nature to become probably the most important organ in your body. Your heart is a large muscle that pumps blood containing oxygen and other important substances to all the organs and cells in your body. In addition, it provides the means to eliminate waste from the body's daily activities.

This guide covers several aspects of heart disease and heart attacks. Learn everything you need to know about heart attacks, their complications, and even the risk factors that make it more likely one day. But the good news is that you can do a lot to reduce your chances of having a heart attack, and you just need to start as soon as possible. In this guide, we'll explore what you can do to get your heart pumping and feeling good.

Everyone wants to make sure they have a strong heart and live a long and healthy life. If you're ready to prevent heart attacks and feel your best, be sure to read this guide and learn the steps you need to take to finally see results and keep your heart strong.

Chapter 1: What Is A Heart Attack Or Myocardial Infarction?

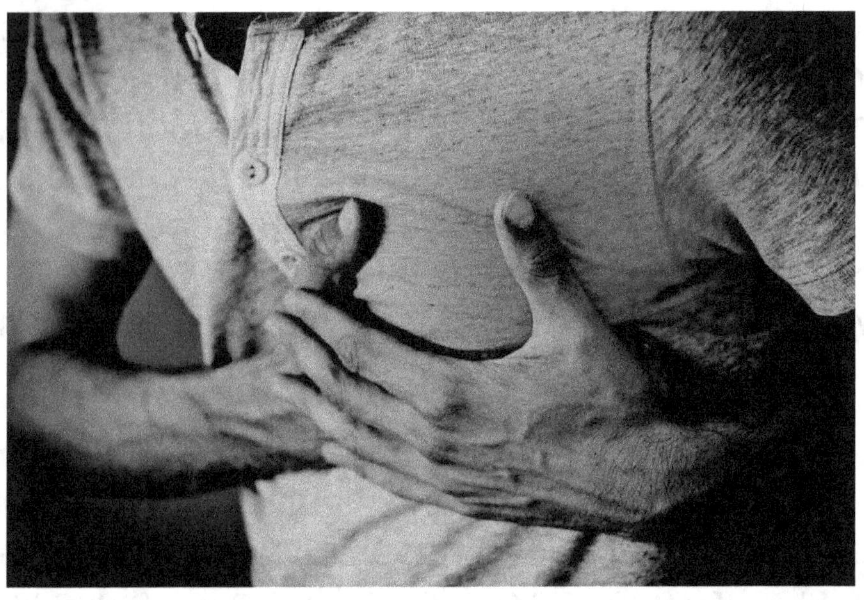

A heart attack occurs when a segment of heart muscle dies or dies due to loss of blood flow. Blood supply is usually lost due to blocked coronary arteries, which supply blood with blood clots to the heart muscle. This condition is also called coronary thrombosis.

When this happens, the person experiences distressing symptoms such as chest pain and electrical instability of heart muscle tissue.

Heart disease is a very general term used to describe all the different disorders and diseases that can affect your heart and how it works. One of the most common causes is oxygen starvation; it is usually the result of a blockage in the arteries that carry oxygen-rich blood from the lungs to the heart. This condition can cause damage to the heart, and if left untreated, necrosis of the affected heart will occur. In other words, heart cells begin to die. This condition is often caused by the buildup of a waxy substance known as plaque.

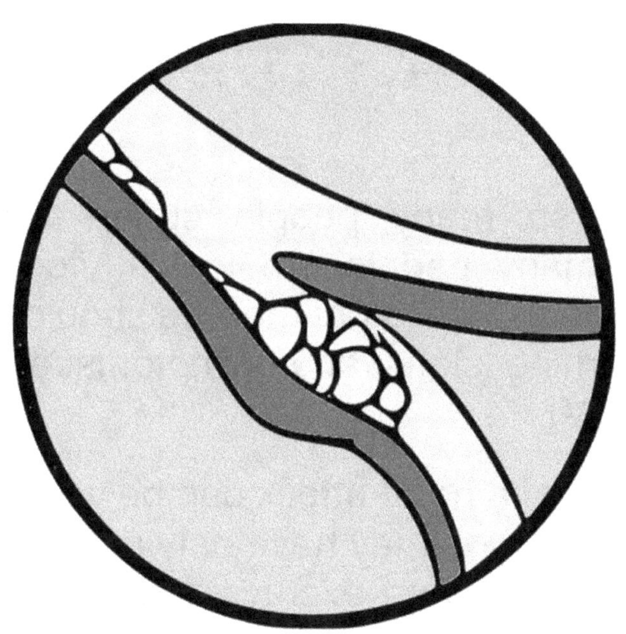

When plaque builds up in your arteries, it can cause partial or complete blockage of the coronary (or heart) arteries. This condition is called atherosclerosis. This restricts blood flow to organs and tissues. If this condition is not treated quickly, the areas of the heart that depend on this artery will die. Previously healthy heart tissue also undergoes fibrosis, forming scars that interfere with the normal function of the heart. Sometimes such a condition disappears from the radar and is difficult to detect. So if you leave it like that for a long time, you will end up with a lot of heart health problems in the long run.

Symptoms Of A Heart Attack Or MI

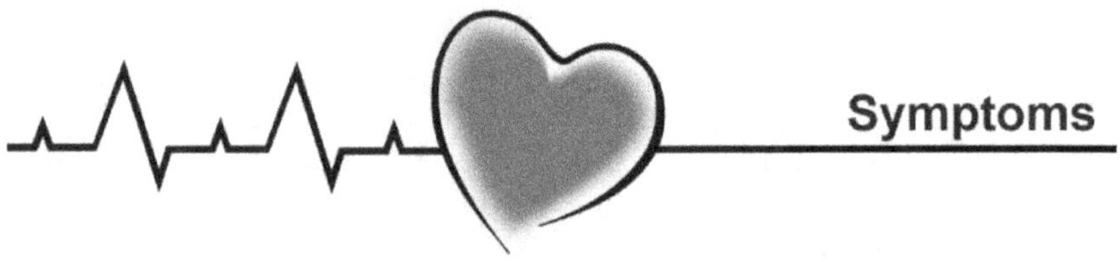

Because so many people suffer from heart attacks, many people are looking for ways to prevent them. But before that, we should learn the early warning signs and symptoms of a heart attack or MI.

Symptoms of a heart attack can be very different. For example, you may have only mild chest pain, while others have excruciating pain. Typical symptoms of a heart attack in men and women are:

> ➢ Feelings of weight, pain, pressure and even discomfort in the chest, under the sternum or in the arm.
> ➢ Discomfort that radiates to the back, arm, throat or jaw.

- ➢ Indigestion, fullness and even choking. Sometimes it can feel like heartburn.
- ➢ Dizziness, vomiting, nausea and sweating.
- ➢ Extreme shortness of breath, anxiety or weakness.
- ➢ Collapse or lose consciousness.

How To Diagnose A Heart Attack Or MI?

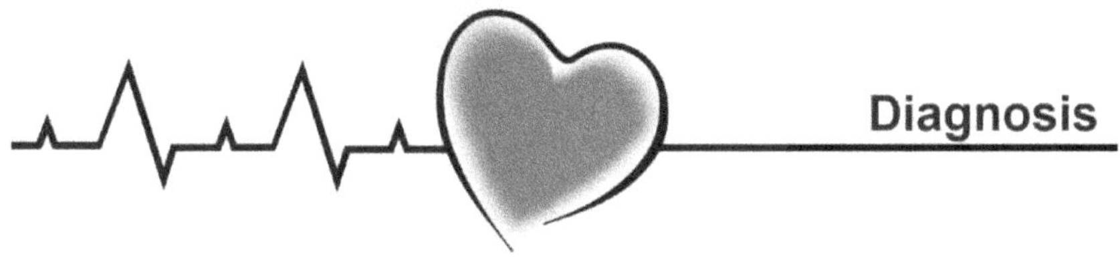

Every year, there are thousands of people who fall victim to a heart attack without even knowing they have one. They act as if nothing has happened because most people are asymptomatic in the early stages of a heart attack until a crisis occurs.

Think of it as a walking time bomb. To identify possible diseases, we look at the symptoms that a person is suffering from. These heart attack symptoms vary from person to person. They can be light or heavy. Mildness and susceptibility also depend on age, sex, presence of risk factors or underlying diseases. For example, people with diabetes tend to have subtle or unusual symptoms.

In any case, if you find that you are having symptoms of a heart attack, you should seek emergency care immediately. When you are dealing with a heart attack, the speed of treatment is extremely important. In fact, the faster the first aid, the greater the chance of survival.

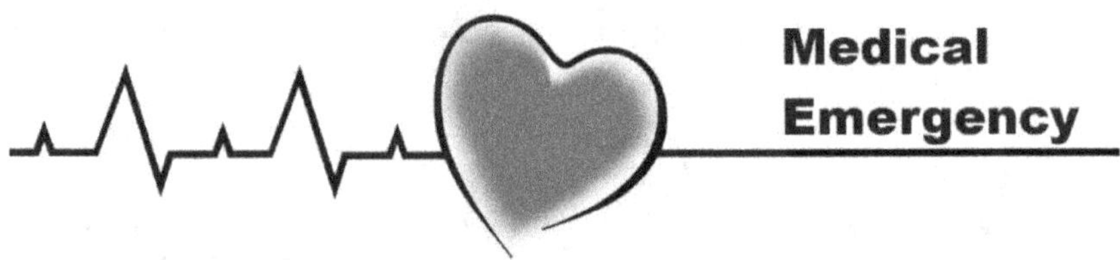

When facing an attack, remember to ask others for help. Do not try to drive or walk yourself to the hospital if you are in excruciating pain, as this will only worsen your symptoms and increase the risk of complications. Ask someone to call emergency heart health service and seek medical attention immediately. Every second counts, and by seeking medical attention early, you can prevent further damage to heart tissue and even survive!

Chest Pain – Cardiogenic VS Non-Cardiogenic

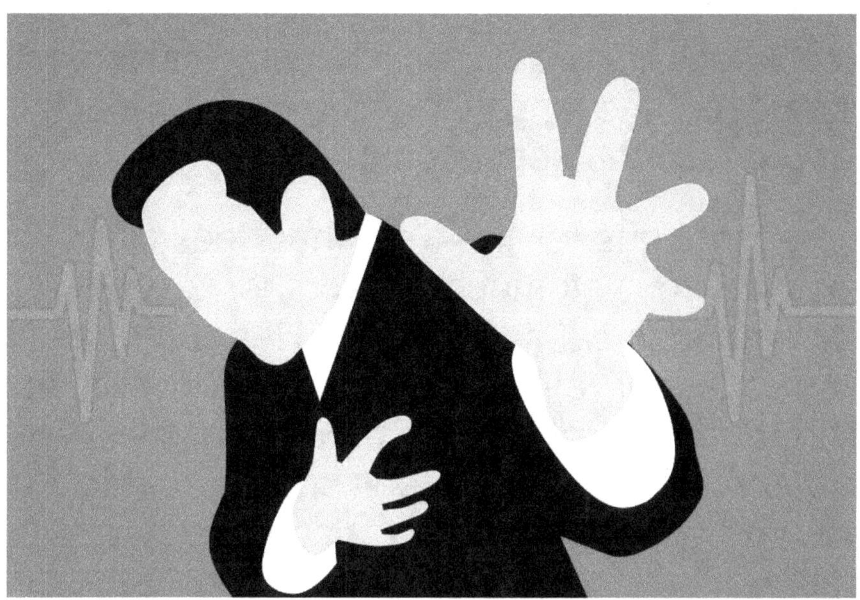

Most people experience chest pain at some point in their lives. This is often due to anxiety, as chest pain is often associated with heart disease. Fortunately, almost all chest pains have little to do with the heart, but it should not be ignored.

Understanding the differences between different types of chest pain can help diagnose heart disease. Pain in the left side of the chest is one of the first symptoms that a person may notice when the disease is detected. The next step is to determine whether the pain is caused by the heart or other factors.

The chest and lung regions are made up of many different structures, all of which can cause pain. The most common pain or tenderness is in the muscles and bone joints around the chest. The lining surrounding the lungs or pleura can be associated with pain when it becomes inflamed or irritated, but the lungs lack the nerve connections that produce the sensation of pain.

The esophagus, or the tube that goes from your mouth to your stomach, is another area in your chest that can cause you pain. Heartburn, as it is often called, or reflux, has nothing to do with your heart, but it can often cause pain that feels like a heart problem. Esophageal spasms, which are also non-cardiogenic, can also occur or cause spasms.

You experience heart or heart-related chest pain more often in the morning. Symptoms include a dull, tight pressure with a burning or pinching sensation. Instead of superficial pain, people usually notice that the pain is coming from deeper areas of the chest. However, describing the location of the pain can be difficult.

Pain can seem to come from all areas, such as the back, neck, head and throat, or even the arms (often the left upper arm). Not knowing where the pain was coming from, people usually described that "the pain came out of nowhere". Chest pain is often caused by some kind of strain, such as carrying a heavy bag, sweeping or digging.

Extreme temperatures during exercise or work can also cause a heart attack. It can also follow after a heavy meal and then physical work. This type of pain usually lasts as long as your physical activity continues, but usually subsides fairly quickly when the activity that caused it is stopped.

Some heart-related pain, such as angina, may be worse when lying down, but standing or sitting and even bending over the area of discomfort can help relieve it.

If you experience this type of discomfort or pain, it is very important to seek medical attention immediately. Other types of chest pain, not related to the heart, most often occur during or at the end of the day. The pain often feels much sharper and is usually in one area that can be easily identified. This type of pain usually occurs without any real warning or specific cause, other than unusual activity.

Heartburn can occur after eating fatty or high carbohydrate foods. These types of pain often come and go quickly, sometimes lasting only a few seconds or minutes, other times they can last for hours. Simple exercises, especially breathing exercises, often help relieve or stop this type of pain. It usually responds well to pain relievers such as aspirin and heat packs.

What Your Medical Professional Will Do?

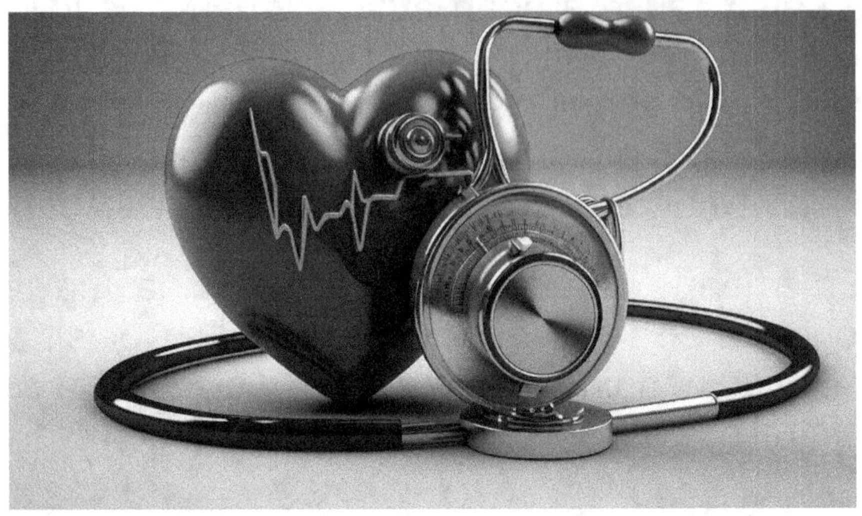

Your doctor will usually ask you several questions, such as your age and gender; your eating habits and physical history. They will take your vital signs such as weight, blood pressure, temperature and may do a test to determine your body fat ratio.

If you're a 25-year-old gymnast or martial arts student who just started lifting weights and taking a bodybuilding class, you might expect your pain to be muscular.

If you happen to be a 56-year-old man who smokes and drinks a lot and does little physical work, strenuous work, also has hypertension, eats mostly processed foods, and has a family history of heart disease; then it's safe to assume that your healthcare professional is looking for a heart-related cause of your pain. This is because all these factors increase the risk of heart attack.

You will probably be asked to do various tests and possibly chest x-rays to find out what your problem is and what is best for you.

If you have determined that your chest pain is caused by a diseased heart, go to the emergency room as soon as possible. Early detection of the cause of the problem can help prevent new attacks and even stop a heart attack. By receiving treatment early, you have the best chance of a full or satisfactory recovery in the shortest possible time.

Chapter 2: Severe Complications Of A Heart Attack

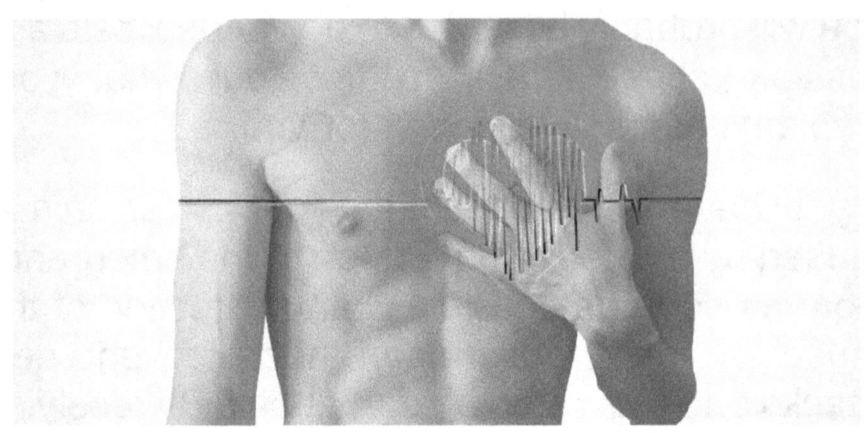

Heart Failure

Heart failure occurs when your heart is unable to pump enough blood around your body to meet all your bodily needs. Heart failure can cause many complications to all the body organs and parts. Areas such as the brain, lungs, kidneys, skin and nervous system can be affected. The veins in the arms and hands, legs and feet, abdomen and neck can also be affected, often becomes swollen. Heart failure can also cause shortness of breath, especially when you're doing physical work.

Valvular Heart Disease

This condition is when the valves in your heart that control the free flow of blood do not work properly. Heart valves ensure that blood flows forward freely and cannot leak backwards. The way a healthy heart works is the same for everyone.

The heart has four chambers, with heart valves at the exit of each chamber. Blood flows through the mitral and tricuspid valves of both the right and left atria into the ventricles. When your ventricles are full, the valves close to prevent blood from flowing back into the atria when the ventricles contract. As the ventricles begin to contract, the aortic and pulmonary valves are forced open. Blood from the left ventricle, after passing through the aortic valve, goes into the aorta and then into the rest of the body. Blood from the right ventricle enters the pulmonary artery through the pulmonary valve.

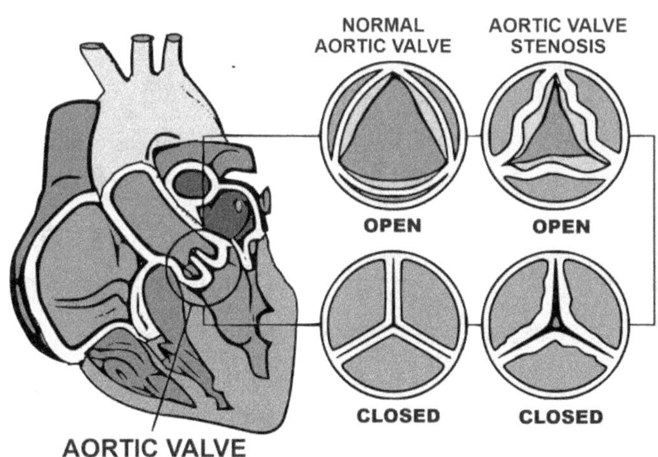

When the ventricles have contracted and begin to relax, both valves are closed. This prevents the backflow of blood. This process is repeated throughout life.

There are two main types of heart valve disease.

Valvular stenosis occurs when one or more valves become narrowed, stiffened, thickened, or blocked. This can cause heart pump failure and lack of blood in various parts of the body. Stenosis can occur in all four heart valves.

Another common type is valvular insufficiency. This occurs when a heart valve does not close or closes properly, causing some of the blood to be pushed or leaked back into the ventricle. When this condition worsens, it forces the heart to work harder to deliver the necessary blood to the body.

Some forms of valvular heart disease are congenital, while others may not be discovered until childhood. Other forms can develop during a person's life. However, the cause is not yet known, but it is definitely related to insufficient nutrition and a sedentary lifestyle. This form of the disease usually affects the pulmonary or aortic valves. Sometimes they may have defective flyers that are incorrectly formatted, incorrectly sized, or incorrectly attached.

Sometimes people are born with bicuspid aortic valve disease; here there are only two leaflets instead of three. As a result, the valves cannot open and close properly and tightly. Acquired valvular disease occurs when the normal valves at birth and early in life have changed or developed complications.

This can be caused by a number of reasons, mainly infections or diseases, including rheumatic fever (caused by an untreated bacterial infection such as strep). Often, if this type of congenital condition is left untreated, it can quickly lead to heart valve disease. Another heart valve disease is known as endocarditis. This happens when harmful bacteria enter the bloodstream and then attack the heart valves. It usually causes pits and tumors and subsequent scarring. These bacteria can often enter the bloodstream through intravenous drug use, dental procedures, surgery, or serious infections.

Another common condition is mitral valve prolapse. It is a disease known to affect approximately 1.5% of the population. This condition causes the leaflets of the mitral valve to move back into the left atrium when the heart contracts. As a result, heart tissue tightens and leaks are most likely to occur in the valves. This condition usually does not become problematic and does not require treatment unless other complications occur.

Another thing that can affect the heart valves are some sexually transmitted diseases, such as syphilis. In addition, high blood pressure and many medications can also cause heart valve damage.

Cardiogenic Shock

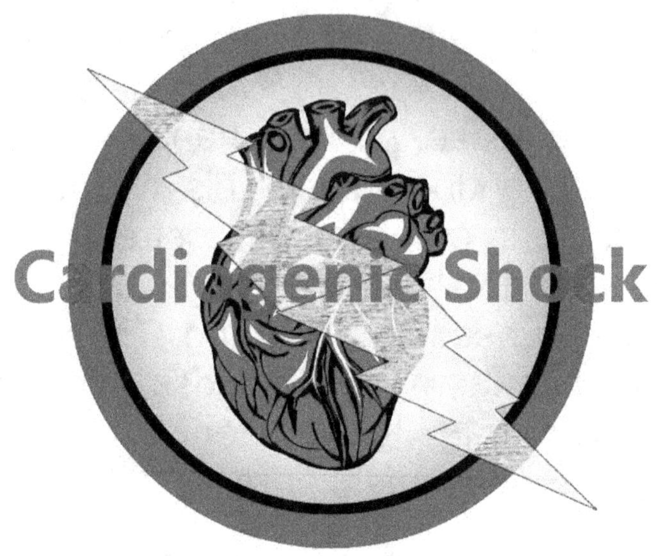

Cardiogenic shock occurs when your heart's pumping action suddenly fails to deliver enough oxygenated blood to your body's organs. Statistics show that about 50% of people who develop this disease will survive if they get immediate help.

This condition is usually caused by damage to the heart muscle. It occurs most often in people who have had a severe heart attack. Only about 7-8% of people who have a heart attack go into cardiogenic shock. When people die of a heart attack, it is usually from cardiogenic shock, not from an actual heart attack. Because of this "shock", the body's blood pressure is dangerously low.

Another type of shock, hypovolemic shock, is when the heart is unable to pump enough blood due to blood loss, usually due to trauma.

Vasodilatory Shock

Vasodilatory shock is when blood vessels suddenly relax, causing blood pressure to drop so low that the pressure is not enough to pump blood to areas that need it. This can be caused by a bacterial infection in the bloodstream or a severe allergic reaction to certain substances. It can also happen when the nervous system is damaged in "shock" for whatever reason, which means that not enough oxygen is getting to their vital organs. They only minutes before the lack of oxygen begins to do damage that usually cannot be repaired. If not treated quickly, it can cause permanent organ damage or death. If you know or think a person is in shock, call emergency heart health service so they can get treatment quickly.

PULMONARY EMBOLISM

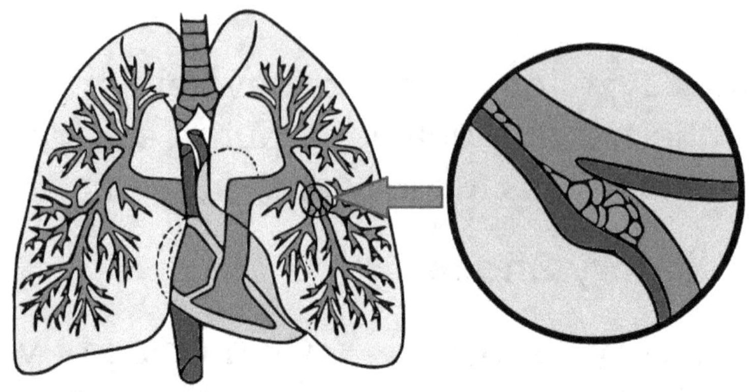

A pulmonary embolism is a blockage of the pulmonary arteries in your lungs. Pulmonary embolism usually occurs when blood clots travel to the lungs from the legs and sometimes other areas of the body (deep vein thrombosis).

Pulmonary embolism can reduce or block blood flow to the lungs, making it life-threatening. With prompt and competent treatment, the chance of death from this condition is greatly reduced. One of the best ways to prevent a pulmonary embolism is to take the right steps to prevent blood clots from forming in your legs. If blood clots form, remove them quickly.

Arrhythmias

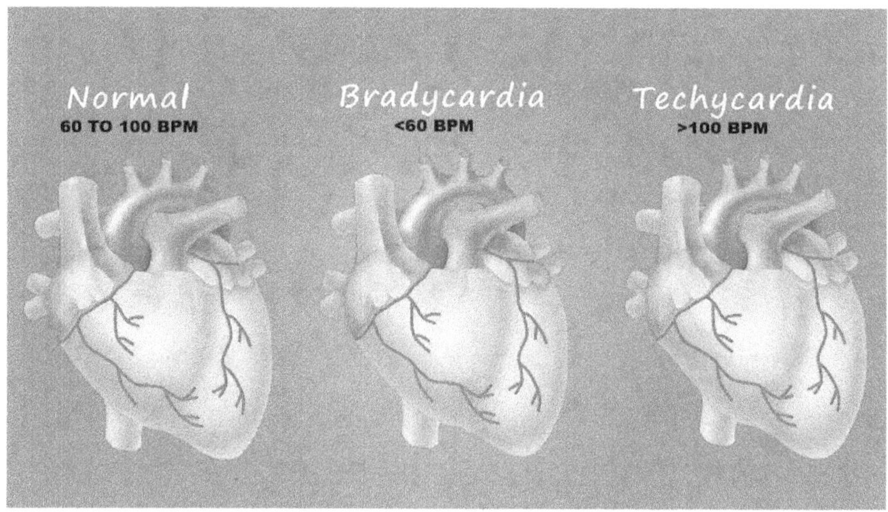

Arrhythmia is the term given to a condition where the rhythm of your heart changes. This can happen if your heart rate is too slow, too fast or irregular. Sometimes the arrhythmia can cause the heart to stop, called "sudden cardiac arrest" or SCA. If not treated immediately, it can cause unconsciousness and death.

Broken Heart Syndrome

This condition is usually triggered by emotional stress and heartache from losing loved ones, falling in love, rejection, repeated anxiety, etc. That's why it's called broken heart syndrome. The most common symptoms of broken heart syndrome are chest pain and shortness of breath; sometimes accompanied by cardiogenic shock or arrhythmia.

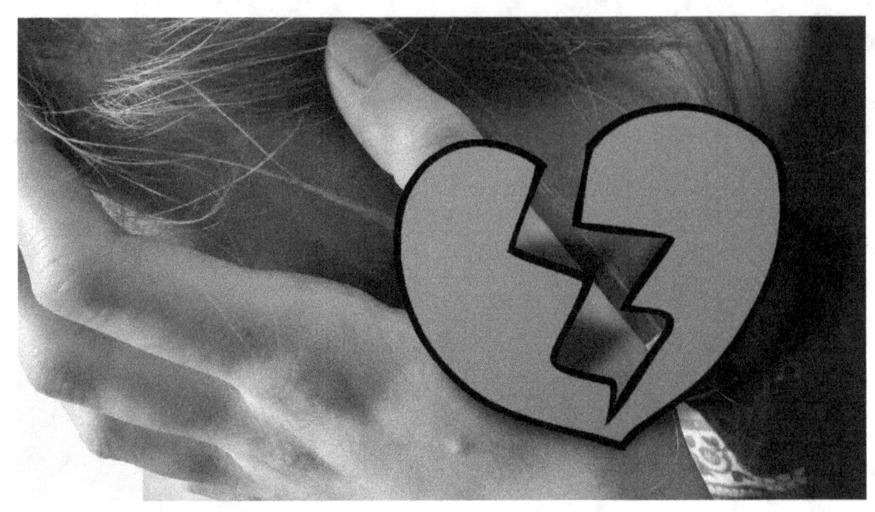

Other symptoms of broken heart syndrome are usually different from those of a heart attack:

> Symptoms appear suddenly after extreme physical or mental stress.
> The results of an electrocardiogram (an ECG is a test to check the electrical activity of the heart) are usually different from those of people who have had a heart attack. For example, those who have had a heart attack in the past will show a deep Q wave on the ECG graph.
> Testing shows no evidence of coronary artery blockage.
> Abnormal movements and a possible balloon are usually present in the left ventricle or lower left ventricle of the heart.
> Recovery time is relatively quick, often in days or weeks, unlike a heart attack, which usually takes a month or more.

As a person ages, blood vessels often harden and lose their flexibility and elasticity over time. Although smoking is believed to be one of the main causes of this condition, the actual cause is still unknown. Chemically derived medicines are likely to be affected by a poor diet or a diet high in preservatives, artificial flavors and colors.

Myocardial Aneurysm

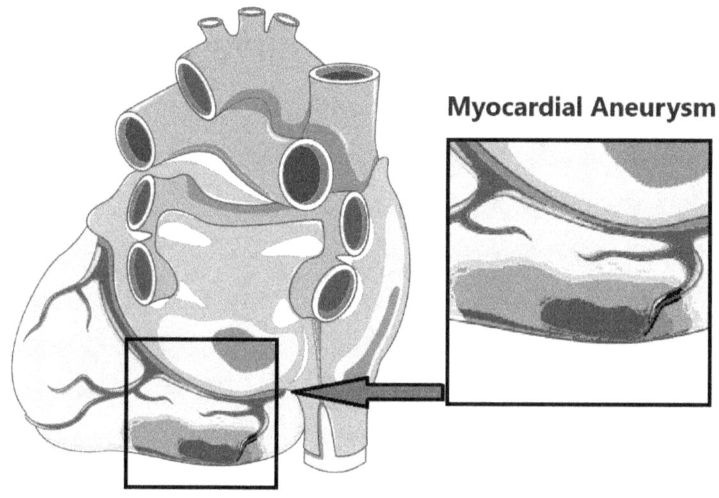

An aneurysm is caused by a weakened blood vessel that causes it to swell and fill with blood. They often occur after a heart attack. They often occur around the base of the septum or in the aorta. This can cause narrowing of blood flow in the body, leading to heart disease. Eventually, aneurysms are covered with scar tissue, which usually prevents them from rupturing.

Ventricular aneurysms usually grow slowly. Common symptoms include fatigue, lack of energy and stamina. Blood clots can form inside some ventricular aneurysms, which can cause serious complications and even death. Death is common when blood clots break up and spread through the bloodstream.

Some aneurysms are congenital, while others are caused by a heart attack. Blood clots that form around them can block blood vessels, causing movement restrictions and tissue death in the limbs, stroke, ventricular aneurysm or arrhythmia.

Chapter 3: How To Provide Emergency Care At The Time Of Heart Attack?

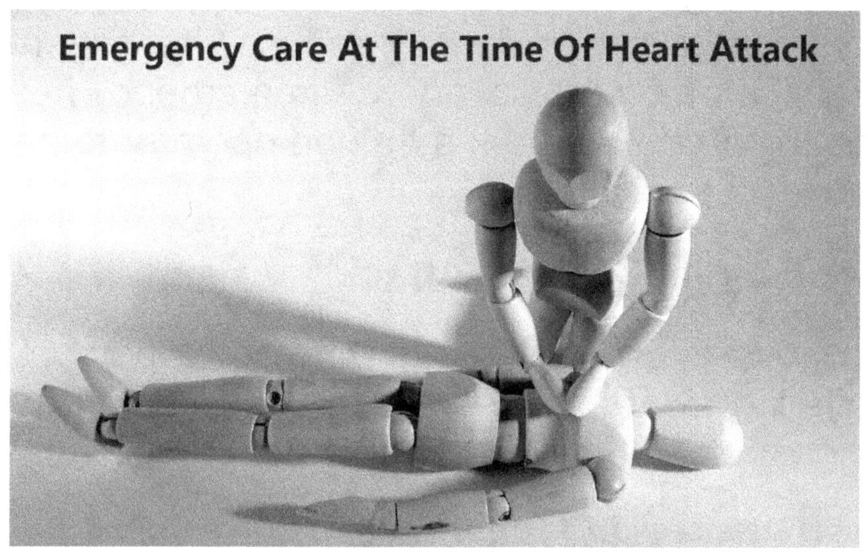

There are often no obvious signs of a heart attack. This disease is usually asymptomatic until the later stages. Early signs of a heart attack are pain or discomfort in the chest and shoulders, fatigue, lack of energy, difficulty breathing, etc.

Complaints can vary from person to person, but when a heart attack actually occurs, they will experience a sharp pain in the left side of their chest for at least 15 minutes. Men and women have different symptoms. For example, women usually do not experience breast pain; their common symptoms are fatigue, sleep disturbances, shortness of breath, indigestion and anxiety disorders.

If you suspect you are having a heart attack, call emergency heart health service right away. Don't wait, because every minute counts. A delay in treatment can significantly reduce the patient's chances of a full recovery. Call emergency heart health service and ask a trained operator to help you.

The 6 Signs Of Heart Attack

So how do you determine whether a person is suffering from a heart attack? Here are the six signs of heart attack that you can take note of.

Heart Attack sign 1: Chest Pain Or Discomfort

For men, chest discomfort is the most common symptom of a heart attack. Usually, they'll experience a tight, heavy, or burning sensation. It can also feel like indigestion or heartburn. This sensation usually begins in the middle of the chest, and then it moves to other areas of the body. This discomfort usually come and go.

Some people experience no pain at all, just discomfort or a dull type of pain, which can grow to be quite intense; others will not have pain just discomfort.

Heart Attack Sign 2: Discomfort Or Pain In Other Parts Of The Body

The symptoms of a heart attack can also manifest in different parts of the body, such as one or both arms, back, stomach, jaw or the neck. Different people, especially women, will experience pain or discomfort in the jaw or back during an attack.

Heart Attack Sign 3: Shortness Of Breath

Feeling short of breath is a common heart attack symptom. It is normal for a person to experience shortness of breath after some physical work or exercise but if this happens when you're resting, it is often a sign of heart attack. It is caused by the leaking of fluid into the lungs. To unusually fatigued women, it can sometimes be an accompanying symptom.

Heart Attack Sign 4: Nausea, Sweating Or Clamminess

Many people, especially women, when having a heart attack will feel nauseous, excessive sweating or clamminess. These symptoms can also be indications of the flu, but if these symptoms occur abruptly or you also have other indications of a heart attack, call the emergency services immediately.

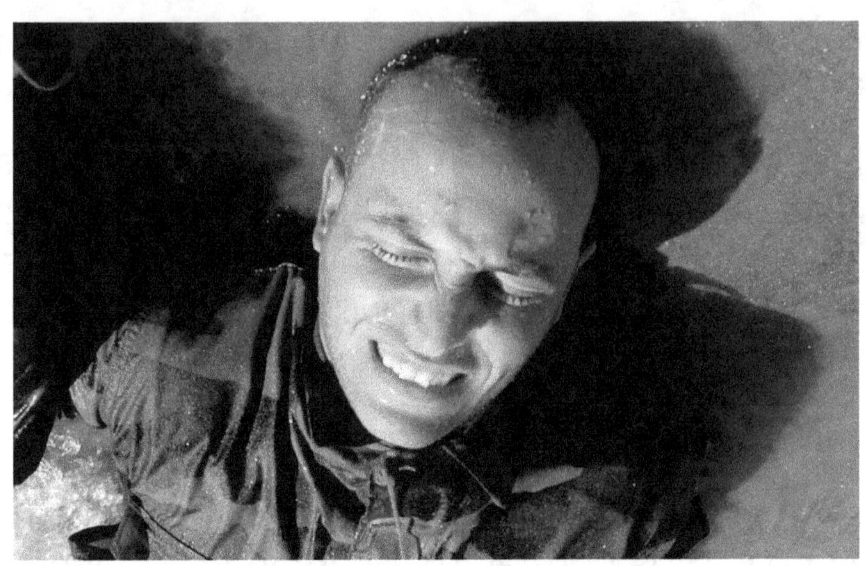

Heart Attack Sign 5: A General Feeling Of Extreme Fatigue Or Weakness

Sometimes, the first complaint you may hear from a heart attack patient is general weakness or fatigue. It might not sound like much, but this is a common indication that most potential heart attack patients experience prior to the attack. But this symptom alone is not enough to diagnose or expect a heart attack as there are too many causes of weakness and fatigue. It can be due to lack of oxygen, not having enough sleep, poor eating habits, anemia, arthritis, and others.

Heart Attack Sign 6: Collapse Or Falling

Often a person with heart attack will collapse or lose consciousness, unlike other chest condition where this rarely happens. Again, if you find someone collapses and lose consciousness, bring him or her to an open area and call for an ambulance right away.

Early Warning Signs Of A Heart Attack

Heart attacks usually warn before they happen (except heart pain). This can often happen days or in some cases months before seizures occur and damage to the heart muscle occurs.

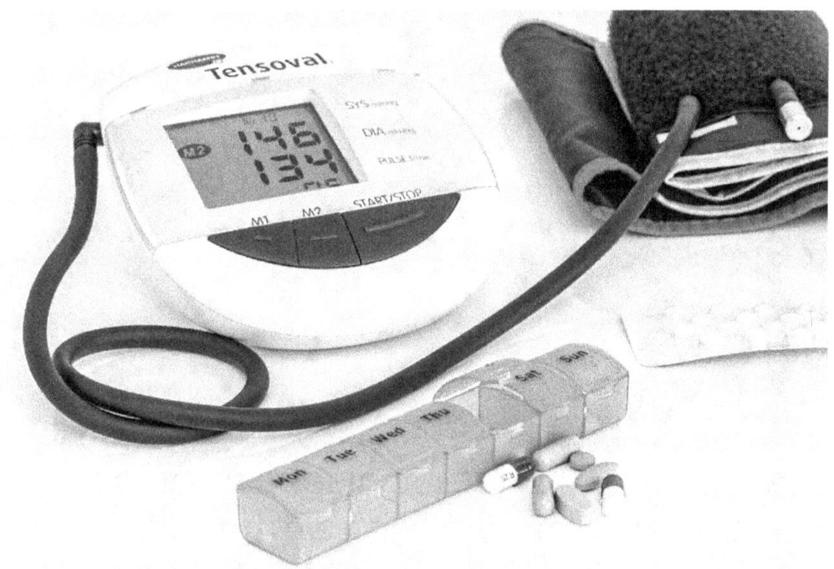

- ➢ High blood pressure is a sign of possible heart disease.
- ➢ Chronic heartburn can be a sign of heart problems.
- ➢ Worsening of cardiovascular disease and shortness of breath.
- ➢ High blood LDL cholesterol.
- ➢ Feeling sick or exhausted before a heart attack.

- ➢ Notifications according to many people feel imminent death before a heart attack. This is quite common and can be associated with depression, which is also a strong indicator of heart problems.
- ➢ Abdominal pain and indigestion are common signs of a heart attack, especially in people over 55 years of age.

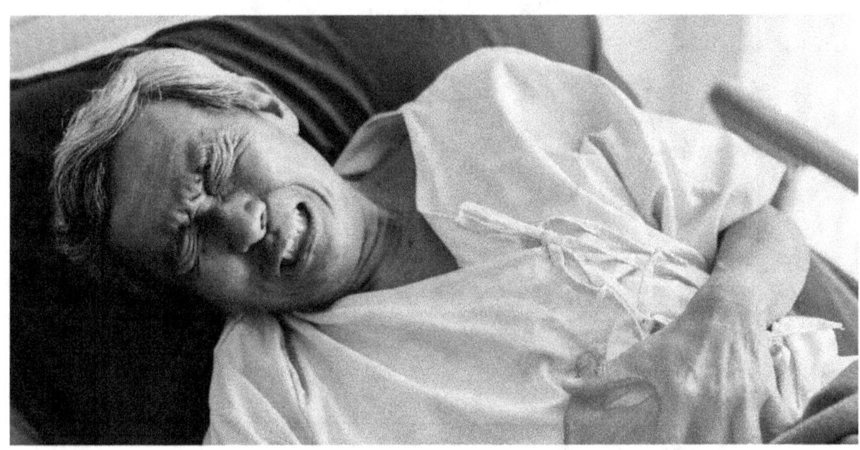

Because many different diseases or conditions have similar symptoms, it can be difficult to tell that you are having a heart attack. Therefore, be sure to pay attention to other symptoms. The more symptoms you find, the easier it is to diagnose a heart attack. For prevention and treatment, it is recommended to visit a health nurse for a routine check-up.

After menopause, some women are more likely to develop heart problems. This is because they produce less estrogen at this stage of life. Therefore, they should change their diet accordingly to reduce the risk of heart disease.

Obesity And Its Effects

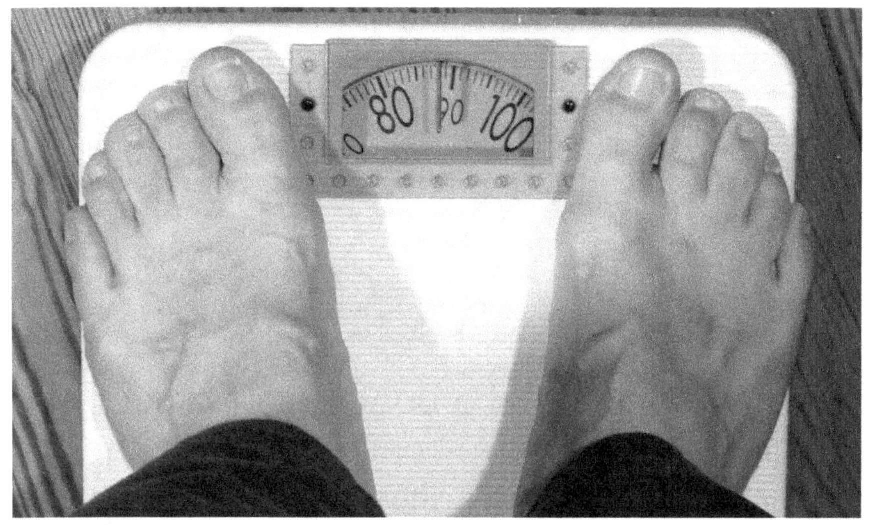

Obesity is a growing global health problem. Obese people are four times more likely to develop heart disease. Additionally, those with a family history of high blood pressure or diabetes have a higher risk of heart disease.

Obesity is now recognized as an inflammatory disease; it is often thought to be a symptom or sign of other human diseases. Not as previously thought, but an eating disorder. Several studies have confirmed that obesity is the main cause of heart diseases and heart attacks.

Poor Diet, The Wrong Foods, Clogged Heart Vessels – Strokes

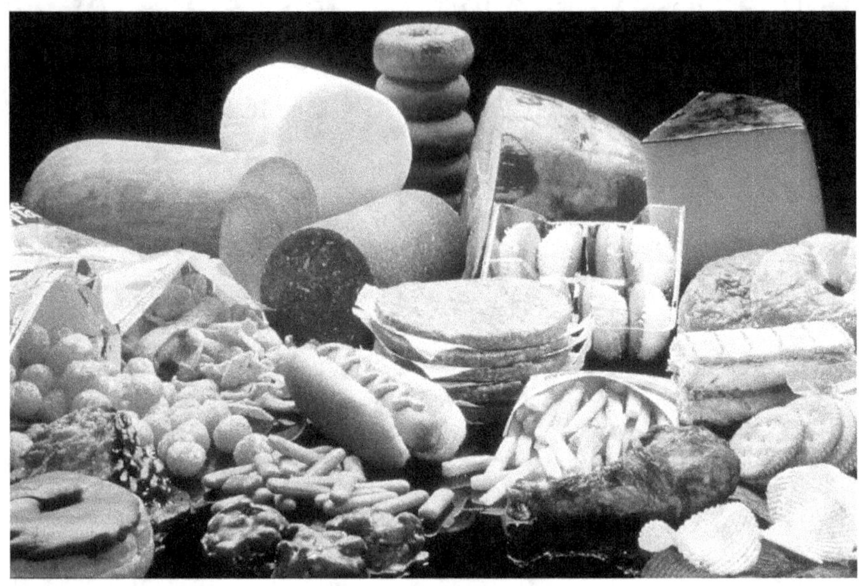

There is no doubt that a poor diet or lack of many essential nutrients is a major factor in the very high incidence of heart disease that has become a reality for many people today.

Due to processing and the synthetic methods used to grow it, a significant amount of its natural goodness has been removed from our food. Refined salt, highly refined grains, high fructose corn syrup and refined vegetable oils are four "poisons" found in most of our diets. Their combination blocks the arteries and blood vessels of the lungs and heart, causing heart disease.

Smoking

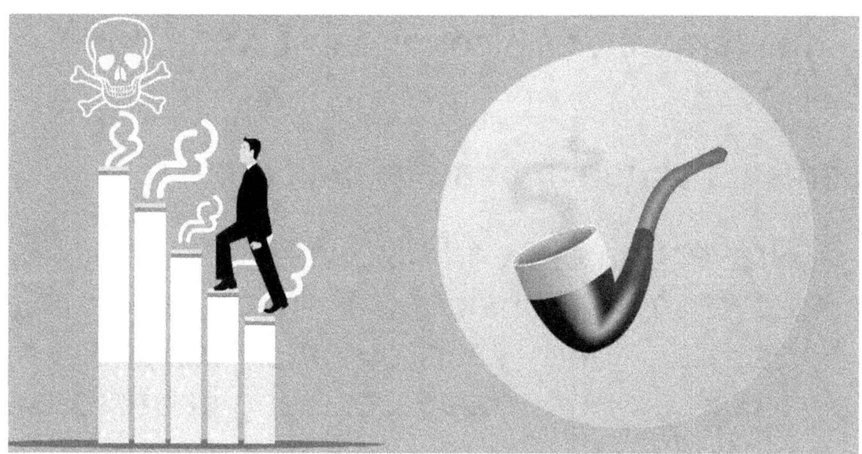

Everyone knows that smoking probably damages your lungs, but many don't seem to realize that it's also a major risk factor for heart disease. In fact, about one in five people die of a heart attack as a result of smoking. If you smoke, you are at least four times more likely to develop heart disease than non-smokers. And the risk is even higher for women who use birth control pills.

Exposure to tobacco is also a risk factor for heart attacks. Nicotine in cigarette smoke reduces the oxygen content of the blood. As a result, the amount of oxygen your lungs can send to your heart is greatly reduced. It also causes high blood pressure and an increase in heart rate due to a compensatory mechanism that your body triggers when there is a lack of oxygen. Nicotine can also damage the inner walls of blood vessels and arteries and also form unwanted blood clots.

Drinking

A small amount of alcohol can contribute to our health.

Examples of health benefits include:

> Prevention of heart disease.
> Lowering your risk of ischemic stroke (which occurs when your coronary arteries are blocked or narrowed, resulting in decreased blood flow).
> Diabetes can lower your risk.

However, doctors do not advise heart patients to drink alcohol under any circumstances. The reason is that 90% of patients who are allowed to drink alcohol cannot control themselves! Instead of drinking a little, they down the whole bottle, especially chronic alcoholics.

Drinking a small amount is beneficial, but more than the recommended amount is harmful.

How does alcohol help prevent heart disease?

Drinking small amounts of alcohol can help raise good cholesterol (HDL) while lowering bad cholesterol (LDL). It also helps stop blood clotting, thins the blood, reduces bleeding and can help prevent heart attacks, but only if used in moderation.

High Cholesterol

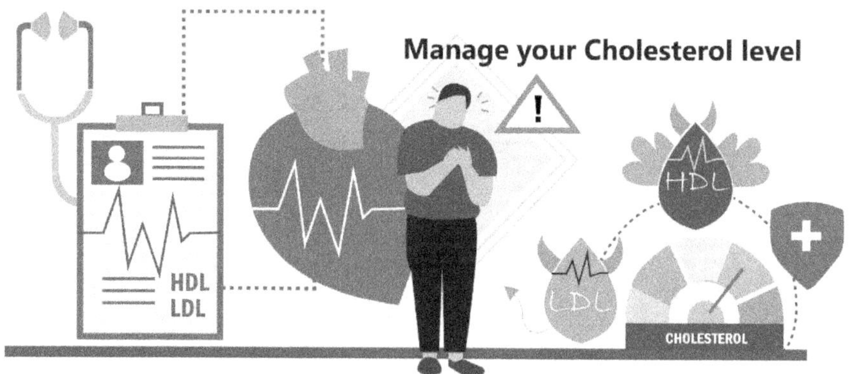

Cholesterol has been blamed for heart disease for years, but now it is known that cholesterol is actually healthy. In fact, it is one of the most important substances produced by the body. After all, the body needs cholesterol to perform its functions. For example, our brain and liver are made of good cholesterol.

Our body can produce its own cholesterol. However, the problem arises when we consume too much "bad" cholesterol, or LDL, or low-density lipoprotein. Eating processed sugars, hydrogenated vegetable oils and excess omega-6 fatty acids causes an excess supply of LDL.

LDL helps transport cholesterol to the areas of our body that need it. If it's too much, the excess can stick to the walls of the arteries, irritate and block them, preventing enough oxygenated blood from reaching the brain, heart and other organs.

Diabetes

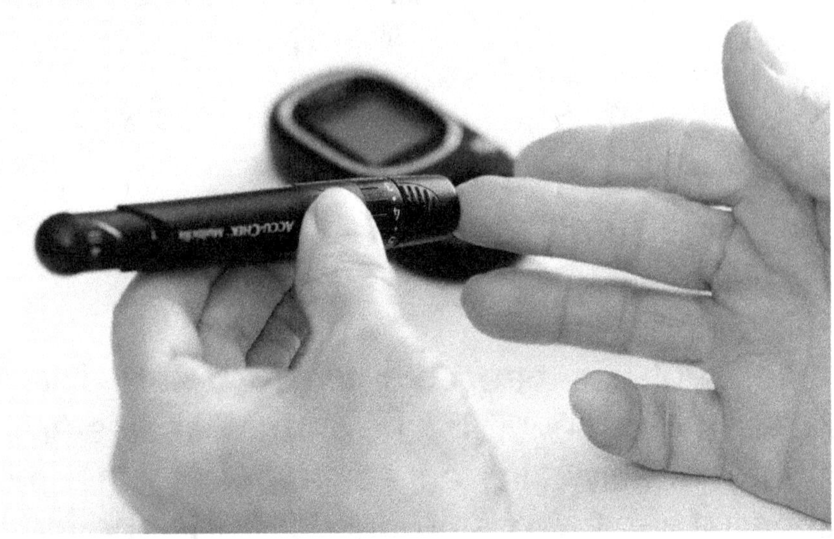

Diabetics tend to have high blood sugar, which over time can damage the blood vessels and nerves that control the blood vessels in your heart. Many people with diabetes can develop heart disease at a young age, and people with diabetes are almost twice as likely to develop heart failure as people without diabetes.

As with all heart diseases, your risk factors can be greatly reduced if you take the right steps to manage your diabetes.

Physical Activity

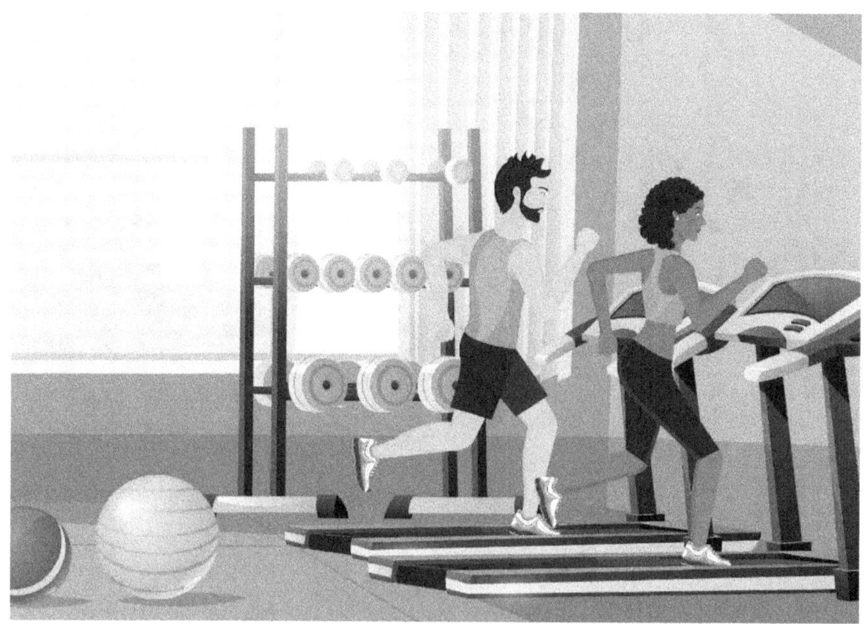

Very little or no physical activity is the biggest cause of heart disease and heart attacks. This is because they cannot burn excess calories, which causes the formation of adipose tissue. The body is designed to perform certain activities every day to keep it flexible, healthy and functioning properly.

When the body receives more food or energy than it needs for a long time, it causes obesity, which can lead to many diseases. The body needs exercise to stay in top shape, which is a great way to exercise for heart health.

Part Two- How To Naturally Have A Healthy Heart

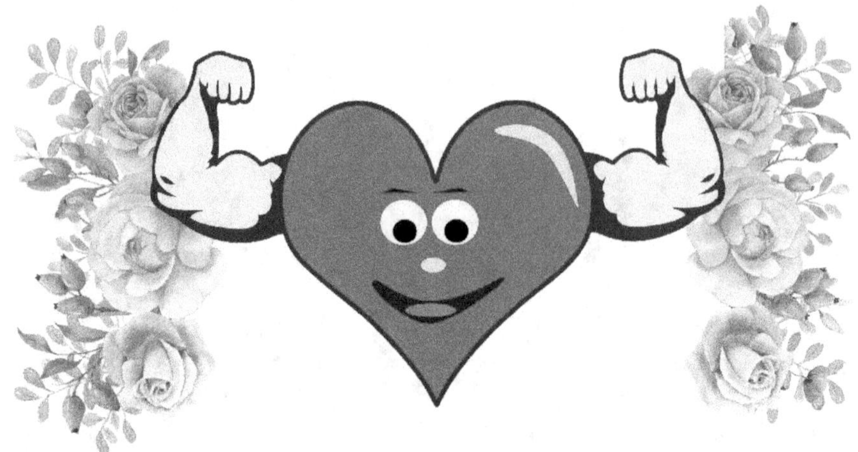

Taking care of your heart is like finding the fountain of youth. It's a no-brainer that if you take care of your heart, you'll live long and healthy. Most people need 7-8 hours of quality sleep a night to maintain a healthy heart, as this is the time for both self-repair and maintaining healthy heart arteries.

If your blood pressure is too high, it can damage the walls of your arteries, causing scar tissue to form and lose elasticity. This condition can make it difficult for oxygen-rich blood to reach your heart and other organs. The harder the heart has to constantly work, the faster it can wear out. That's why it's important to maintain a healthy blood pressure.

Pay attention to your diet and avoid processed foods as much as possible. At the same time, do not forget to do as many physical exercises as possible.

The human heart works best when it produces high-quality, clean fuel, which means fresh, healthy organic food and minimally processed foods.

Also choose healthier beverages such as fruit juices or plain water instead of soft drinks to improve your overall health. Try to balance your work and home life. Spend more time with family, friends and loved ones. This exercise is good for mental and physical health. To maintain a healthy heart, check your vital signs regularly.

Chapter 5 Make Your Heart Healthy And Strong With These Lifestyle Changes

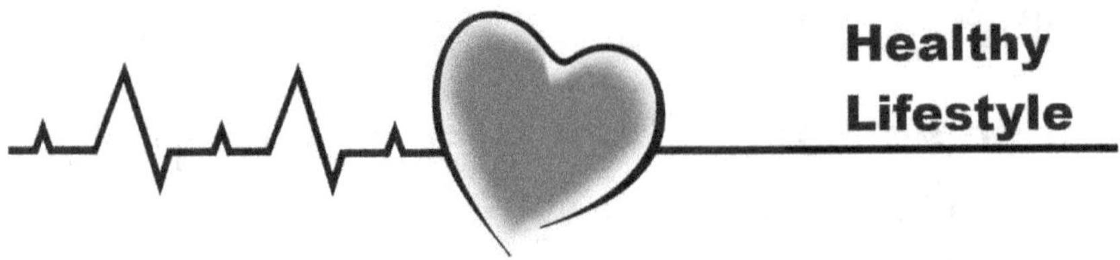

There comes a time in everyone's life when we have to make a decision and commit to healthy lifestyles. They often notice that their body is starting to break down, are in the final stages of an illness or are experiencing the pain of losing a loved one to ill health. These situations are often a turning point in their lives where they finally decide what is best for them and their family.

It is always better to live a healthy life, full of vitality, youth and vigor, than to live a sick life, constantly relying on health care. Our environment plays an important role in our heart health. Therefore, if your lifestyle is not conducive to health, for example, you live in a highly polluted area with poor hygiene and health services, the best option is to move elsewhere.

Diet: The Importance Of A Healthy Diet

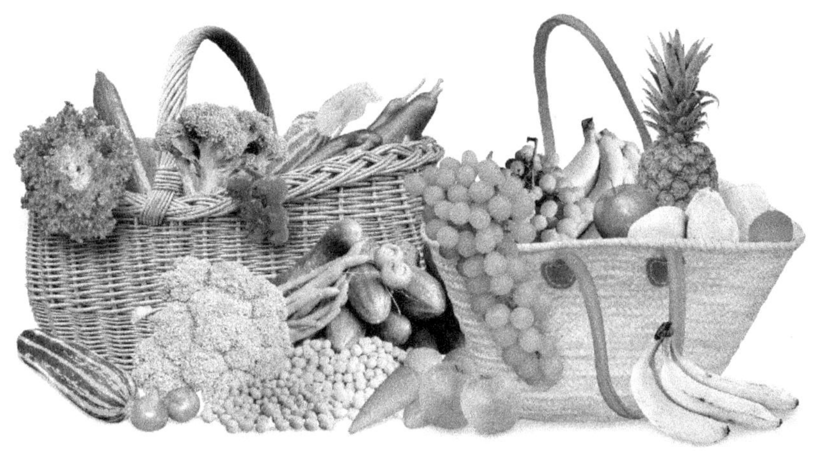

Our body and heart form a very complex organic living machine, but far more advanced than any human can create. But like any machine, it needs the right fuel and lubrication to run. Have you heard the saying that "Your body is your vehicle on this journey of life"? That's why you should respect your body more than anything else. Consider putting cheap vegetable oil in your new car or trying to fill the tank with cheap, dirty old fuel.

So why do you do this to your body, you can always buy a new car, but you can't get a new body (well, maybe a new heart, but what a hassle and expense). It definitely makes sense to use only the best fuels for your body! Of course, by fuel I meant your diet. Choose only foods that will benefit your health, not destroy your body.

Exercise - The Best Heart Exercises

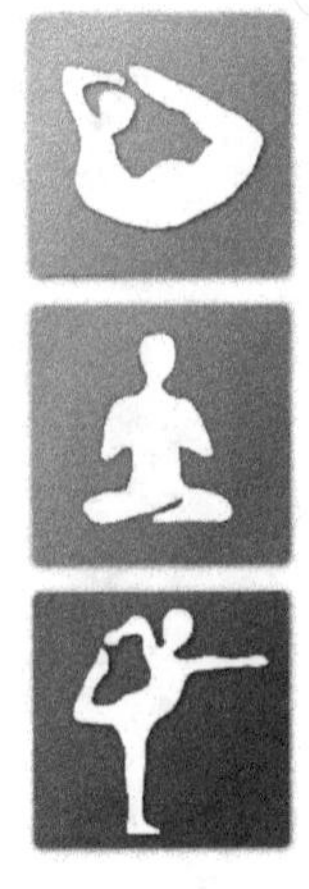

Do best heart exercise recommended by doctor

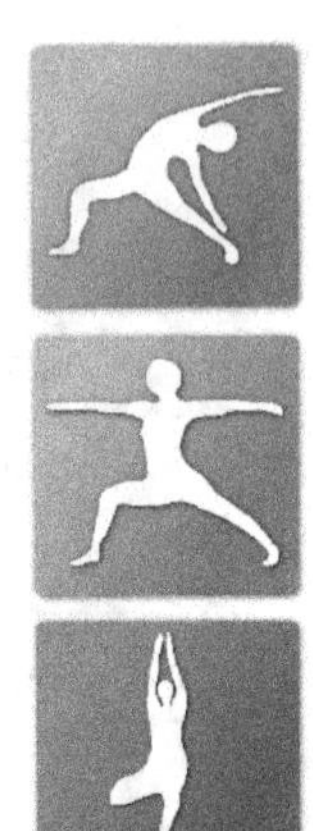

So what is the best and most effective exercise to prevent heart disease? Research shows that high-intensity exercise with slightly longer active recovery periods is not only good for your heart health, but it can also help with weight loss, diabetes and improve your overall fitness.

This can be done by walking for 3 minutes at your normal speed and then walking briskly for 1 minute. By constantly raising and lowering your heart rate with simple, high-intensity exercises, you can improve blood vessel function, burn more calories, and also improve the body's detoxification functions.

Another great cardio workout is a full-body, non-impact sport like tennis or squash, swimming or rowing, kickboxing or other martial arts. All of these involve the use of many different muscles, so train your body well without overloading any one area, but making your heart work hard to deliver them all. With slow intervals, you can also create your ideal workout that matches your current fitness level.

Core exercises such as push-ups and squats help strengthen the core muscles and give the body a good foundation. People who are active all day tend to be healthier than those who exercise 30 minutes to an hour a day and are sedentary the rest of the day. But remember that not all exercises are good for the body. For example, jogging or running long distances on hard surfaces is probably the worst form of exercise, even though they strengthen the heart. This is because this type of endurance training wears out the body quickly and stresses the joints in the long run, especially without a pair of comfortable shoes or proper running techniques.

It is also not recommended to do exercises for which no training or warm-up has been done. This will only lead to unwanted injuries and even trigger a heart attack due to the adrenaline rush. If you like a workout routine, stick with it and improve it, adding instead of changing something you might not like.

Stress Reduction

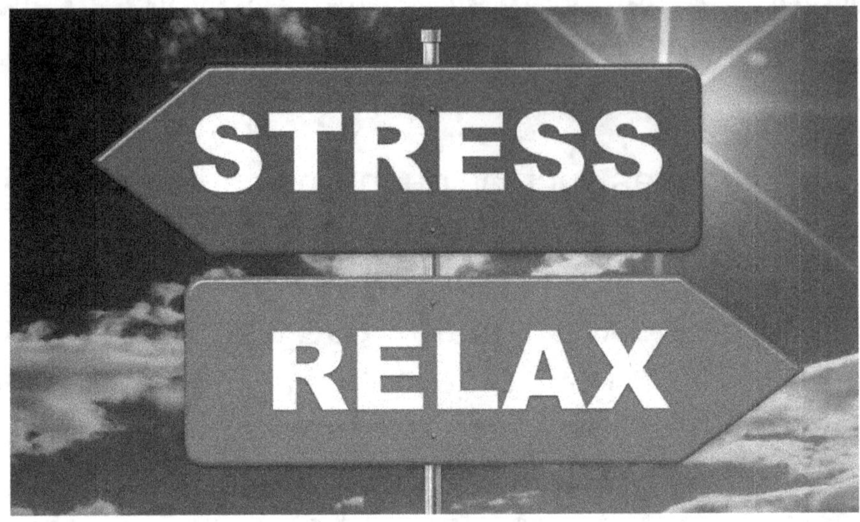

Many studies show that psychological factors can influence heart disease and possible heart attacks. Anxiety, anger, depression, hostility and social isolation can affect the risk factor for heart attack.

Work stress and financial stress can increase the risk of a heart attack by 50%. After the terrorist attacks of September 11, 2001 on U.S.A, it was found that people who experienced high levels of stress immediately after the attack were twice as likely to develop high blood pressure and three times as likely to develop heart disease in the following two years. Similar results have been observed after major earthquakes and other natural disasters.

Environmental Conditions, Clean Air And Water

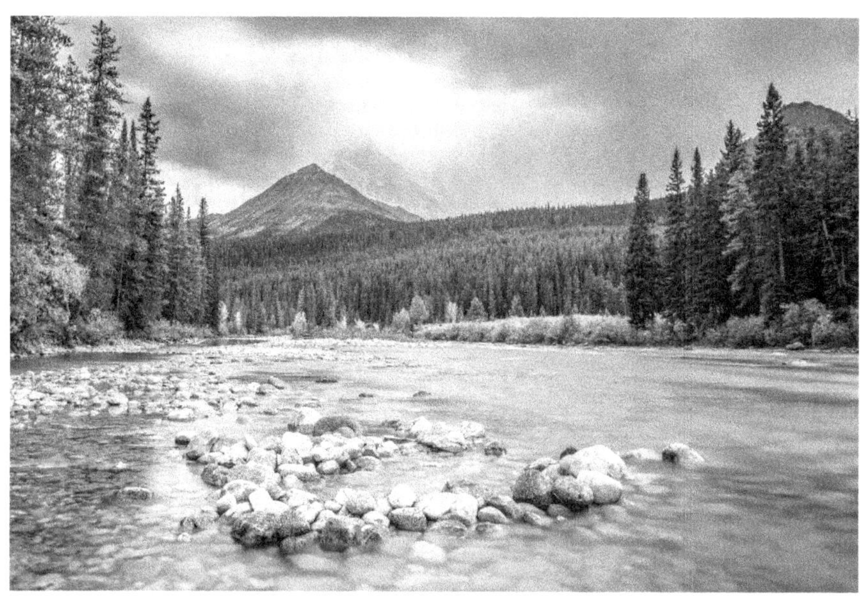

Water and air pollution contribute significantly to heart disease and stroke in humans (a stroke is like a heart attack to the brain). Being indoors too often may not be as safe as you think because indoor air is polluted.

Pollution comes from a variety of pollutants, such as fumes from household cleaners, wood stoves and fireplaces, cigarette smoke, fumes from cleaning products, paint thinners, pesticides, insecticides and carbon monoxide.

Exposure to low levels of CO (carbon monoxide) can cause heart arrhythmias, chest pain and irregularity in cardiovascular patients, making exercise difficult. CO in indoor air can come from indoor furnaces, dryers, gas water heaters, space heaters, furnace vents, and wood stoves.

There is evidence that several minerals commonly found in drinking water can promote heart disease or worsen its symptoms. Exposure to lead, arsenic, fluoride and chlorine is clearly associated with heart disease.

Chapter 6: Healthy Heart Remedies

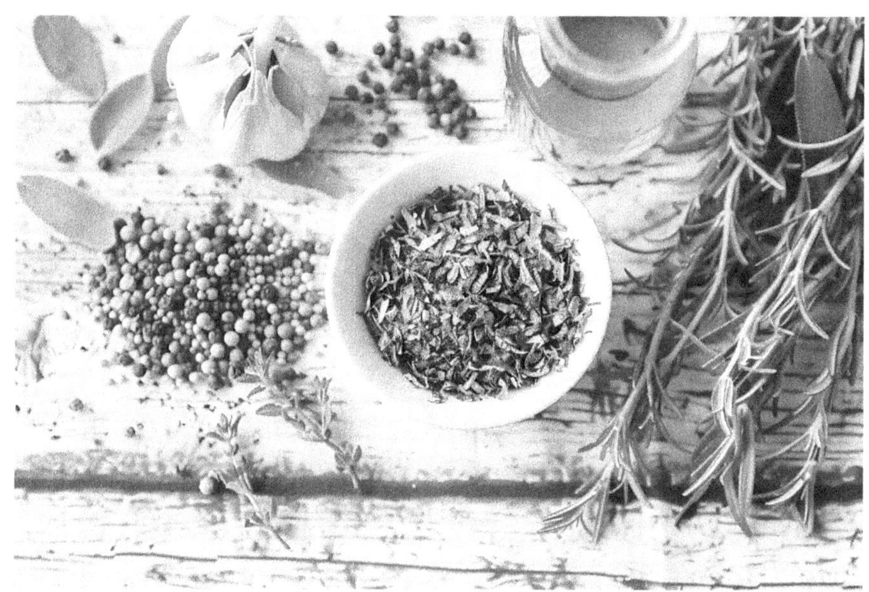

Many natural remedies use various herbs and supplements to treat and prevent heart disease. Atherosclerosis, the hardening of the arteries, is a common cause of heart disease. This disease occurs mainly in western countries. On the other hand, atherosclerosis is relatively rare in third world countries due to lifestyle, traditional diet and availability of herbal medicines. Most importantly, they are free of processed food chemicals and toxins that can harm heart health.

Coenzyme Q10, or ubiquinone, is a compound that helps our cells obtain energy from food. This compound is often lacking in our diet. Although coenzyme Q10 is produced naturally in our bodies, its amount decreases sharply as a person ages or cholesterol levels drop. Therefore, by adding coenzyme Q10 to your daily intake, you can ensure that your body has enough nutrients to keep your heart and cells healthy.

If you don't get enough magnesium and potassium in your diet, taking these supplements can help control your blood pressure and improve heart function. As you may or may not know, salt goes way back in human history. It plays a central role in the development of human civilization as well as in the public health policy of the last centuries. Although salt has been considered a valued ingredient for thousands of years, it has been demonized in the last century. Today it is even called one of the most harmful substances in the human body.

However, recent studies have shown that although salt intake affects heart health, it still plays an important role in maintaining a healthy heart and optimal health. In fact, too little salt can cause various diseases and harm your body in the long run. Therefore, we should consume salt in moderation to improve our health.

Where do we get salt?

Natural, unrefined sea or rock salt is an excellent source of minerals.

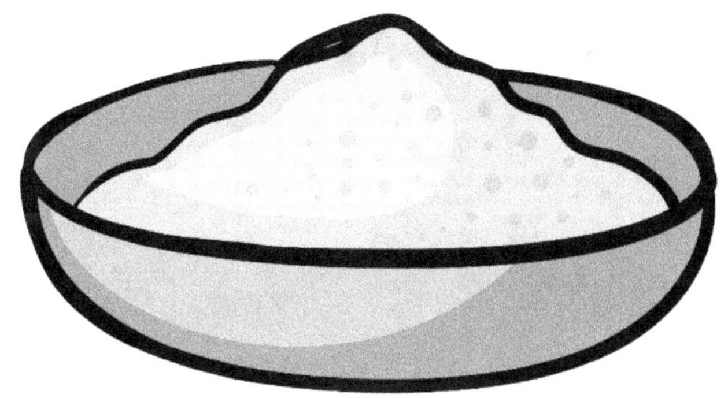

Sea salt is the best source of salt we can find to enrich foods with lots of minerals. Today, due to the lack of nutrient-rich soil, it is difficult to find even a trace of healthy minerals in our food. So by adding a variety of sea salts to our diet, we get much-needed minerals from Earth's oceans.

But not all salt is good for our health. In fact, table salt, which is mined from underground salt deposits, is highly processed and harmful to our health. Processed table salt has been stripped of its natural minerals and often contains additives that prevent caking.

The health benefits of ocean minerals are only available when you choose an all natural sea salt that is "worth its salt". Not to mention the incredible flavor it can bring to your best dishes.

Fish Oil And Other Supplements

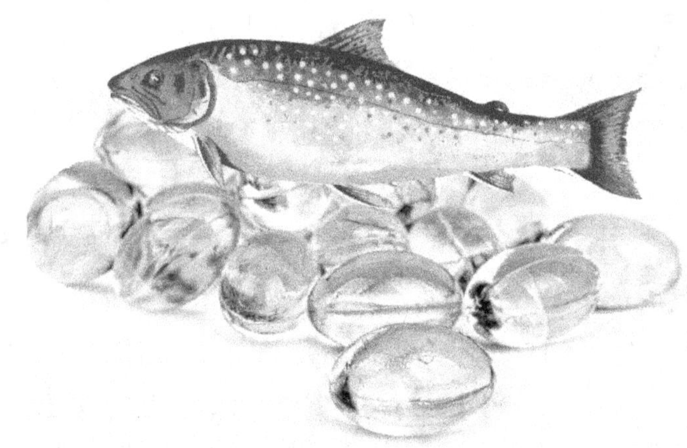

Many supplements, such as fish oil, are often of low quality and can be harmful. This is due to the extraction process used, which causes them to oxidize. Before buying or taking supplements, it is important to get access to quality. A good healthy diet usually fulfills all the needs of the body.

The only time supplements are necessary is if your diet is deficient or certain health conditions cause you to be deficient or deficient. Most supplements are safe and some offer real health benefits, but their use can come with risks. Some are also anti-nutrients; they prevent the body from absorbing nutrients.

Omega-3 fatty acids are essential nutrients found in naturally grown plants, free-ranging, wild-fed livestock and sea-caught fish. They are usually found in nature in an ideal 50/50 ratio for heart health with other natural fats such as omega-6 fats.

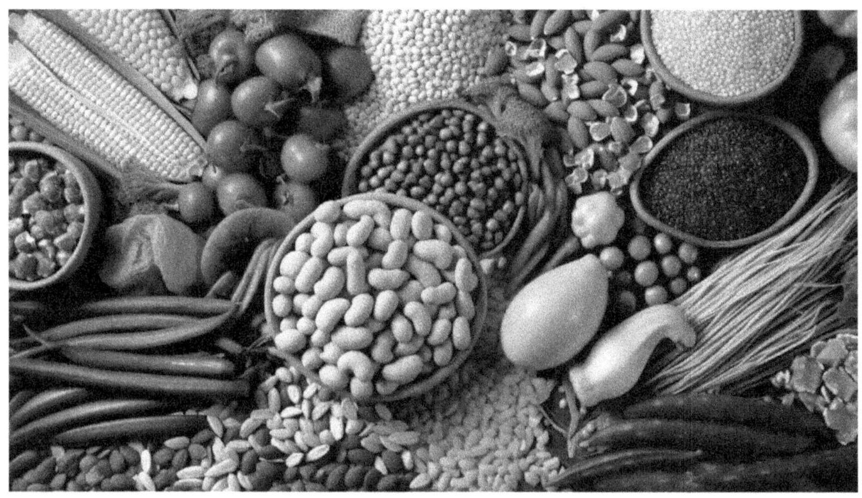

Livestock, such as eggs, dairy and shellfish, lack many essential nutrients when raised in feedlots or factory farms without natural feed or natural sunlight. They lack omega-3 fats and contain many unhealthy fats.

So unless you are using a free range organic diet, it is highly recommended that you supplement your diet to meet your daily nutritional needs.

Vitamins And Their Importance

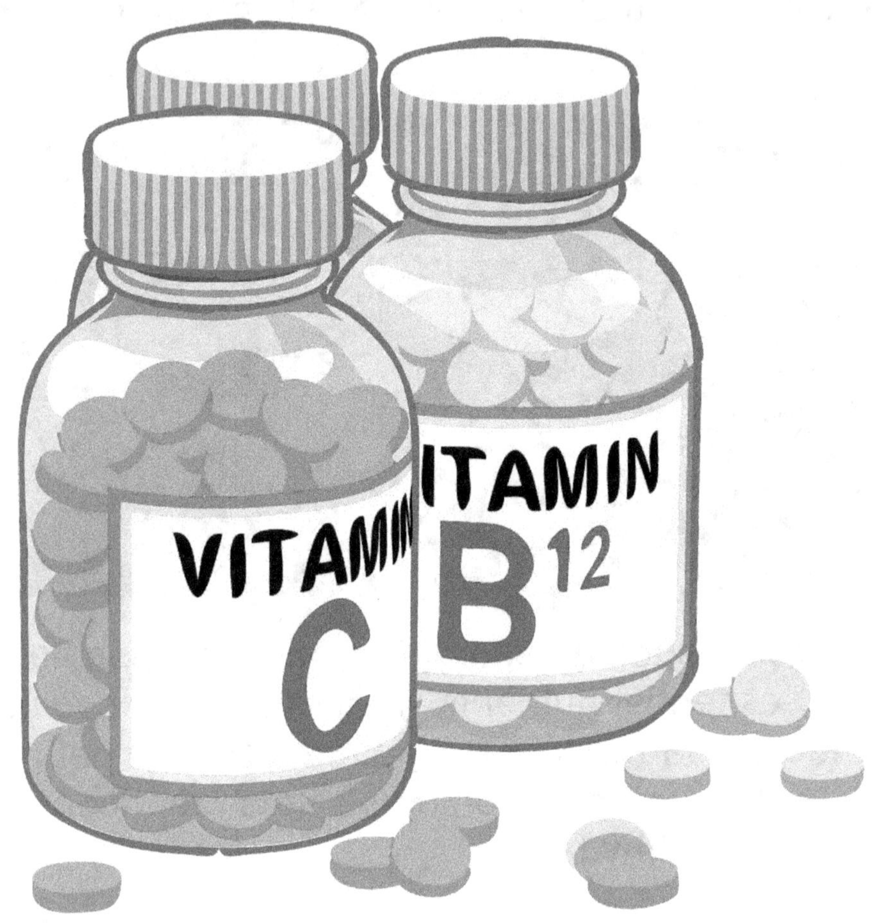

Health experts believe that vitamin C is undoubtedly one of the safest and most essential nutrients for the human body. If you take a daily dose of vitamin C, your body will get the same effect as walking. Simple exercise, such as walking, can stimulate the protein Endothelin-1, which causes small blood vessels to constrict. Research shows that people who take a daily 500 mg, release dose of vitamin C can suppress the activity of Endothelin-1 as much as those who walk regularly.

Vitamin B9, also known as folic acid, is one of the water-soluble vitamins. It is one of the most important vitamins that you should include in your daily nutritional needs. Our liver acts as a storehouse of vitamins.

Our body uses the necessary amount of vitamin from this store every day. The excess amount of vitamins is then automatically removed from our body through the excretory system. Vitamin B9 helps perform one of the body's most important functions, which includes everything from the formation of red blood cells to the production of vital energy.

In addition, vitamin B9 also offers health benefits such as a protective barrier against cancer, stroke, heart disease and birth defects. Other benefits include building muscle, increasing hemoglobin and preventing mental and emotional breakdowns. Vitamin B9 is found naturally in Asparagus, Broccoli, Brussels sprouts and Lentils.

Enzymes In Foods

Enzymes are essential for every cell in our body because they are organic biological catalysts that initiate, promote and accelerate biochemical reactions.

Metabolic enzymes in the blood break down protein-based defenses against viral parasites, bacteria and fungi. They are cleansing agents that fight chronic inflammation and prevent most diseases, including heart disease.

Our body produces many enzymes; millions every day, but we still need a lot of fresh enzymes from fresh foods.

Antioxidants

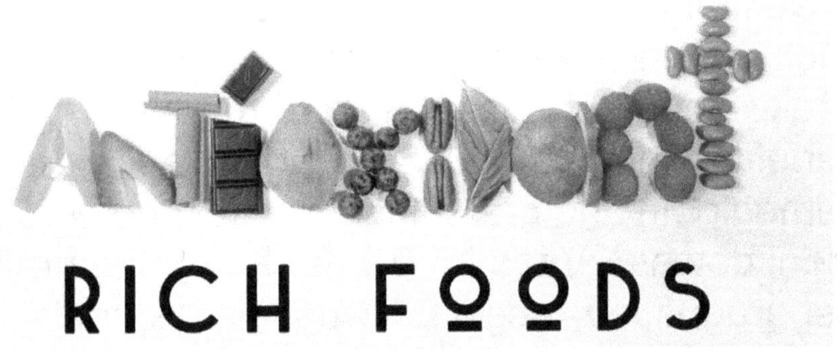

Antioxidants are molecules that donate electrons that help maintain the integrity of your cells. Antioxidants help prevent cholesterol oxidation. In fact, oxidized cholesterol is the cause of death.

Although oxidation is one of the body's normal processes, it can be life-threatening if too much oxidized cholesterol is produced.

Why this?

This is because, unlike other oxidation products, oxidized cholesterol is usually mistaken for bacteria by our natural immune system. So your body does everything it can to remove oxidized cholesterol from the body, which causes inflammation of the artery walls. As a result, it can cause atherosclerosis or even heart disease.

There are many well-known antioxidants, but one of the most well-known is vitamin E. Study after study has shown that vitamin E is a powerful antioxidant that can help prevent and even treat free radical damage.

Factory Farming VS Organic Foods

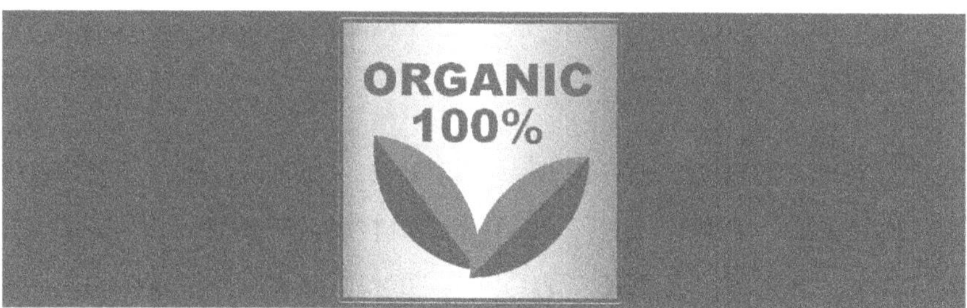

Have you heard of the term "factory farming"? It's a modern term that refers to an "unconventional" approach to farming that focuses on high-stocking conservation. They are able to achieve this goal by adopting modern technology to boost animal growth, increase production and reduce livestock mortality.

Modern society, especially business owners and investors, agree that factory farming is the way to go for modern agriculture. Factory farming was also seen as one of the main innovations and probably solved countless problems, producing large volumes of production and lower costs. On the other hand, there are those who oppose it and claim that factory farming does more harm than good to both our health and the environment. Animal activists also protest animal cruelty in factory farming.

What is the truth?

After years of careful monitoring and extensive research in the agricultural industry, it has been discovered that most factory farms use poor quality ingredients and questionable processing methods.

On the other hand, there is the "organic agriculture" method. This term refers to a more natural, less toxic approach to growing and producing agricultural products. For example, organic crops must be grown without modern agricultural chemicals such as GMOs

(Bioengineered genes), synthetic pesticides, sewage sludge and oil-based fertilizers.

Organic animals must not be injected with growth hormones, antibiotics or animal by-products. Organic animals must be raised on organic feed and given the opportunity to move outside. Anything less cannot be called "organic".

Therefore, organic products are much more nutritious and less toxic to our bodies. Eating more organic foods and less processed foods can improve health and retain more nutrients.

Detox - The Real Story

Our bodies, if given the raw materials needed are very good at detoxing themselves. People who have a healthy wholesome diet and refrains from indulging in too many processed foods (a small amount of processed food is not ideal, but the body can deal with it if not overloaded) will enjoy renewed energy and heart health.

Meditative Cures, Reflexology And Mindfulness

Psychological risk factors such as anxiety and depression are clearly factors that can have significant effects on the heart. Stress can influence and increase risk factors for heart disease and high blood pressure (BP), especially when accompanied by physical inactivity and excess weight.

According to the latest clinical findings, meditation can significantly reduce the risk of heart disease, stroke and even death by approximately 50%. They found that deep breathing and intense relaxation can be more effective than the latest super drugs in preventing or even treating heart disease.

The ultimate goal of meditation is to find "balance" in our bodies. Although it may seem incomprehensible and difficult to understand to most of our society, meditation has been shown to balance our biomarkers in the body. These biomarkers are also known as hormones and neurotransmitters.

When you experience stress or pain in any part of your body, it is usually caused by hormonal changes and neurotransmitter imbalances. An effective remedy for this situation is meditation.

This practice has helped countless patients regulate their biomarkers.

Why is meditation so effective?

The secret lies in practicing mindfulness.

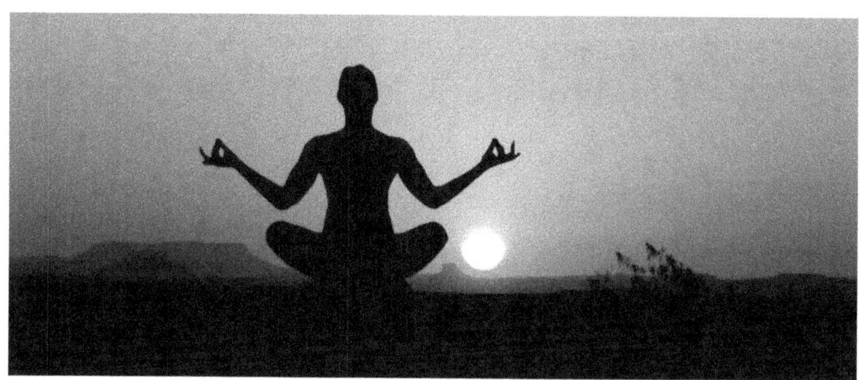

Mindfulness is a term that refers to the ability to focus your awareness on the present moment and everything around you, both internally and externally.

One of the keys to mindfulness is to always be in the moment. Be present with your thoughts, feelings and behaviors without judging them. The practice of non-judgment is really the essence of staying calm and present.

The benefits of mindfulness are limitless. Studies have shown that people who regularly practice mindfulness are more likely to live longer, have healthier hearts, stronger immune systems and are less likely to be obese.

Another alternative treatment for heart health is reflexology. This method appeals to those looking for a non-invasive treatment. In fact, some people may even find reflexology quite relaxing and therapeutic. You don't need to visit a reflexology center to benefit, because you can easily apply these self-relaxation techniques to your hands and feet at any time if you know how to do it right.

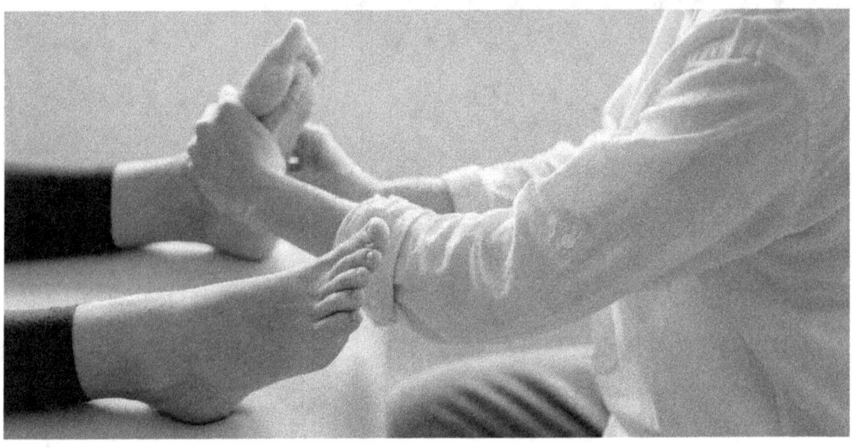

Reflexology helps maintain the balance of mind and body, keeping them in a state of homeostasis so that the body can function optimally. By applying pressure to specific pressure points on the body, trained reflexologists are able to correct faulty posture and bring your body back into a natural state of balance.

Applying pressure to certain pressure points can stimulate muscles, tissues and even cells in any part of the body. These pressure points are also called hand and foot reflexes.

Different pressure points affect different parts of the body. To relax and stimulate the heart muscles, pressure points are located in the reflexes of the legs, which indirectly also stimulates the work of the colon and pituitary gland.

Super Foods For Heart Health

There are many foods that have properties that can dramatically help with heart health problems, mainly because they are very rich sources of nutrients and compounds that naturally clean blood vessels, clean and eliminate inflammation and strengthen the immune system.

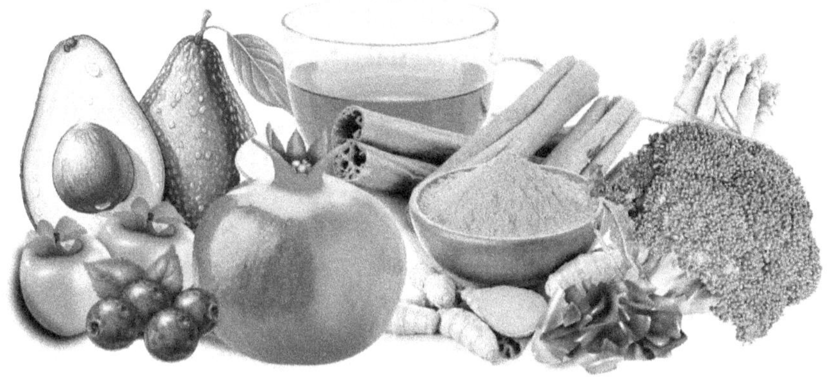

- Avocados contain a lot of healthy fats and eaten regularly, their compounds can normalize and stabilize blood cholesterol, keep arteries clean and remove blood clots.
- Asparagus has been found to be a very effective blood purifier, it can lower. blood

pressure and slow the formation of blood clots. It is full of vitamins B1, B2, C, E and K.

- Pomegranate contains an impressive amount of antioxidants that help protect the membranes of the arteries; they also promote the production of nitric oxide, which allows a person's blood to flow more freely through the blood vessels.
- Turmeric reduces inflammation and hardening of the arteries and helps keep them clean and reduce blood clots.
- Persimmons are a very good source of polyphenols and antioxidants, both of which help lower bad cholesterol (LDL) and triglycerides. They also help normalize blood pressure and clean the arteries.
- Spirulina helps regulate blood fat levels, normalizes lipid levels and contains essential amino acids that help improve the immune system.
- Cinnamon is able to lower harmful cholesterol levels and clear plaque, so it cannot accumulate in arteries and blood vessels.
- Broccoli helps prevent calcium build-up in the arteries and helps lower blood pressure and normalize cholesterol.
- Cranberries are thought to reduce the risk of heart disease in most people by up to 40%.

They are high in antioxidants that help increase HDL and lower LDL.

- ➢ Green tea contains large amounts of catechins, which help slow the absorption of cholesterol and improve blood lipid levels, helping to clear blockages in the arteries. Green tea also helps cardiovascular health and boosts a person's metabolism.

Daily Heart Health Precautions: A Step-by-Step Guide

Maintaining your heart is vital for enjoying a long, healthy life. Heart disease continues to be one of the top causes of death across the globe, yet many types can be prevented or controlled through lifestyle adjustments and daily routines. Below is a detailed step-by-step guide outlining daily precautions you can implement to safeguard your heart and ensure it operates at its best.

1. Start Your Day with a Healthy Breakfast

The day should begin with a nutritious breakfast that promotes heart health. A well-balanced meal aids in managing blood sugar, cholesterol, and blood pressure levels. Choose whole grains, such as oats or whole-grain bread, which offer a high fiber content. Complement this with heart-friendly foods like:

Fruits (e. g. , berries, apples, bananas)

Nuts (almonds, walnuts)

Healthy fats (avocados or olive oil)

Lean protein (eggs, Greek yogurt, or plant-based substitutes)

Steer clear of processed, sugary cereals or pastries, as they can lead to elevated cholesterol and blood sugar levels, heightening the risk of heart disease.

2. Engage in Regular Physical Activity

Physical exercise is among the most effective methods to safeguard your heart. Consistent physical activity enhances cardiovascular health by lowering blood pressure, minimizing cholesterol levels, and boosting circulation. Strive for a minimum of 30 minutes of moderate exercise (such as walking, cycling, or swimming) most days of the week. Include strength training (utilizing bodyweight exercises, free weights, or resistance bands) at least twice each week. Incorporate activities that elevate heart rate like brisk walking or jogging to support heart health. Exercise further aids in maintaining a healthy weight and alleviating stress, both of which are crucial for cardiac health.

3. Eat a Heart-Healthy Diet

Your dietary choices significantly influence heart health. The focus should be on foods that enhance cardiovascular well-being while avoiding those that could be detrimental. Consume heart-healthy fats like omega-3 fatty acids present in fish (salmon, mackerel), flaxseeds, and chia seeds. These fats can reduce the risk of heart disease by diminishing inflammation and enhancing cholesterol levels. Restrict saturated fats (found in red meat, full-fat dairy, and processed food items) and avoid trans fats (common in numerous baked goods and fried products). These fats can elevate bad cholesterol (LDL) and reduce good cholesterol (HDL). Boost fiber intake through abundant fruits, vegetables, whole grains, and legumes. Fiber assists in lowering cholesterol and sustaining healthy blood pressure levels. Minimize salt consumption by preparing meals at home more frequently and steering clear of processed foods. Excess sodium can elevate blood pressure, which may increase the risk of heart disease. Incorporate a diverse array of colorful vegetables and fruits for antioxidants that protect the heart against oxidative stress and inflammation.

4. Stay Hydrated

Staying hydrated is essential for the overall performance of your body, including heart function. Dehydration can force your heart to exert more effort to circulate blood throughout the body. Drink water consistently throughout the day to keep hydration levels in check. Limit consumption of sugary beverages, such as sodas, juices, and sweetened drinks, as these can heighten your chances of obesity and heart disease. Include herbal teas (like green tea) that are high in antioxidants and beneficial ingredients for cardiovascular health.

5. Track Your Blood Pressure

Elevated blood pressure, or hypertension, is a significant risk element for heart disease. Over time, untreated hypertension can harm the blood vessels, resulting in heart attacks, strokes, and various cardiovascular problems. Monitor your blood pressure consistently, either at home or during appointments with your healthcare provider. Maintain a healthy blood pressure level, ideally around 120/80 mmHg. If it is high, collaborate with your doctor to create a strategy to reduce it. Decrease salt consumption, handle stress, and exercise frequently to manage your blood pressure effectively.

6. Handle Stress

Ongoing stress can adversely affect your heart by increasing blood pressure and leading to unhealthy behaviors like overeating, smoking, or excessive drinking. Learning to handle stress is crucial for heart health. Utilize relaxation methods such as deep breathing, meditation, or mindfulness. Exercise consistently to release endorphins, which can enhance mood and alleviate stress. Allocate time for hobbies and activities that bring you happiness, whether it's spending time with relatives or engaging in creative activities. Ensure you get sufficient sleep (7-9 hours) to allow your body to recuperate and cope with stress more effectively.

7. Obtain Sufficient Sleep

Sleep is vital for heart health, as it enables your body to rest, heal, and repair itself. Poor sleep quality or lack of sleep can elevate the risk of heart disease. Strive for 7-9 hours of sleep each night to support overall cardiovascular health. Develop a sleep schedule by going to bed and waking up at the same time on a daily basis. Set up a sleep-conducive environment, which includes a cool, dark room and steering clear of screens before bedtime.

8. Refrain from Smoking and Limit Alcohol Intake

Smoking is among the primary risk factors for heart disease. It harms blood vessels and decreases oxygen levels in the bloodstream. Likewise, excessive alcohol use can raise blood pressure and contribute to obesity. Stop smoking or avoid starting. Seek support groups or use smoking cessation tools if necessary. Restrict alcohol consumption to moderate amounts (up to one drink daily for women and two for men).

Excessive alcohol can elevate blood pressure, harm the heart, and lead to unhealthy weight gain.

9. Maintain a Healthy Weight

Being overweight or obese considerably heightens your risk for heart disease by increasing blood pressure, cholesterol levels, and blood sugar levels. Keeping a healthy weight is essential for your heart. Monitor your weight routinely and aim for gradual weight loss if you are overweight. Prioritize nutrient-dense, low-calorie foods to sustain a healthy weight. Engage in regular exercise and make minor, sustainable adjustments to your diet to assist in losing excess weight.

10. Comprehend Your Family Background and Secure Regular Check-ups

Genetics affect your likelihood of developing heart disease, so it is crucial to understand your family background. Being informed about the prevalence of heart disease in your family can help you take proactive steps to decrease your risk. Consult with your physician regarding your family background so they can provide customized advice. Arrange consistent appointments with your healthcare provider for check-ups and screenings. Regular assessments of cholesterol, blood pressure, and blood sugar levels will allow you to track your heart health and detect potential issues early.

11. Foster Positivity and Social Connections

Maintaining a positive outlook and having meaningful social relationships is essential for mental and emotional well-being. Experiences of isolation and depression may elevate your risk of heart disease. Engage in social activities that enable you to be with others, whether that involves spending time with family and friends or participating in community events. Nurture gratitude and focus on the uplifting aspects of life to help lessen stress and enhance heart health.

Conclusion

Thank you for purchasing this guide. I hope you will enjoy this book and benefit greatly from it. As a general rule, the overall health of our body begins with taking care of our heart. When you take care of your heart, you take care of the rest of your body.

The decisions you make about your diet and lifestyle will ultimately affect your heart health and overall well-being. Not only that, it also affects your family. If you follow a diet that consists mainly of processed foods, you are poisoning your body with empty carbohydrates and chemicals. Also, if you are inactive most of the day and lead a sedentary lifestyle, you can expect to have serious health problems at some point in your life and this can ultimately shorten your life.

On the other hand, if you live a healthy lifestyle, take sensible precautions with your diet and exercise. then you can expect to live a long and healthy life without heart problems and many other chronic health problems that plague most people. That way you can enjoy your golden years in relatively good shape.

* 9 7 9 8 3 3 3 0 3 8 5 0 0 *